Ketogenic Diet For Diabetics

Is This the Ideal Diet for Diabetics?

Ron Kness

Sneak Peek

Due to the exponential increase in diagnosed cases of Type 2 diabetes, awareness of diabetes in a general sense has become widespread. In spite of this, there is no shortage of misinformation and misunderstanding about diabetes, including similarities and differences among the different types.

Depending on the type, diet can play a significant part in cause, prevention and especially management of the condition. A person suffering from diabetes, by necessity, must become more aware of the food they consume.

Different diets and dietary protocols become much more than fleeting choices, they are truly lifestyle choices.

The ketogenic diet is one which has gained acceptance by many sufferers and medical practitioners. However, it is also a subject which has become a victim of misunderstanding.

This book explains what the ketogenic diet is and how it can be of help to many diabetics. It also has chapters on ketoacidosis, which will be very helpful in clearing up common misunderstandings between that dangerous condition and ketosis, which is a natural and mostly beneficial result of ketogenic dieting.

According to the American Diabetes Association, in 2015, over 30 million Americans had diabetes. This staggering number equates to about 9.4% of the population.

And even worse, diabetes was the 7th leading cause of death in the United States in 2015.

In recent years the ketogenic diet has received a lot of attention. Originally created to help combat epilepsy in pediatric patients, the ketogenic diet gained much more popularity as people noticed dramatic weight loss.

It has also been shown to help with chronic pain issues, fibromyalgia, arthritis, IBS, cholesterol, and blood pressure, to name a few. So, why wouldn't the ketogenic diet be beneficial for those people battling diabetes?

In fact, it might just be the ideal diet for some diabetics. Let's take a closer look …

Ketogenic Diet for Diabetics

Sneak Peek.. 2

Disclaimer 7

Introduction 8

Is the Ketogenic Diet Safe for Diabetics?.................................. 10

What is Diabetes? 11

Can the Ketogenic Diet Help? 11

Keto and Type 2 diabetes.. 13

Keto and Type 1 Diabetes 13

Can the Ketogenic Diet Help Reverse Kidney Disease in Diabetics? 14

Ketogenic Fuel vs. Glucose Metabolism 15

Could Ketogenic Fuel Be the Answer?................................... 15

A Study on Mice.. 17

What Does This Mean for Humans 17

Long Term Effects of Following the Ketogenic Diet 19

The Good 20

The Bad... 20

The Ugly.. 21

The Future 22

What Happens When You Have Diabetic Ketoacidosis?............ 24

Keto + Acid + Osis 24

The Perfect Storm 24

Treatment for DKA.. 27

Difference Between Ketosis and Diabetic Ketoacidosis............ 28

Ketosis Defined 29

Ketoacidosis Defined 29

Signs and Symptoms 29

Risk Factors 30

How Are the Two Diagnosed and Treated? 30

Conclusion 33

About the Author 34

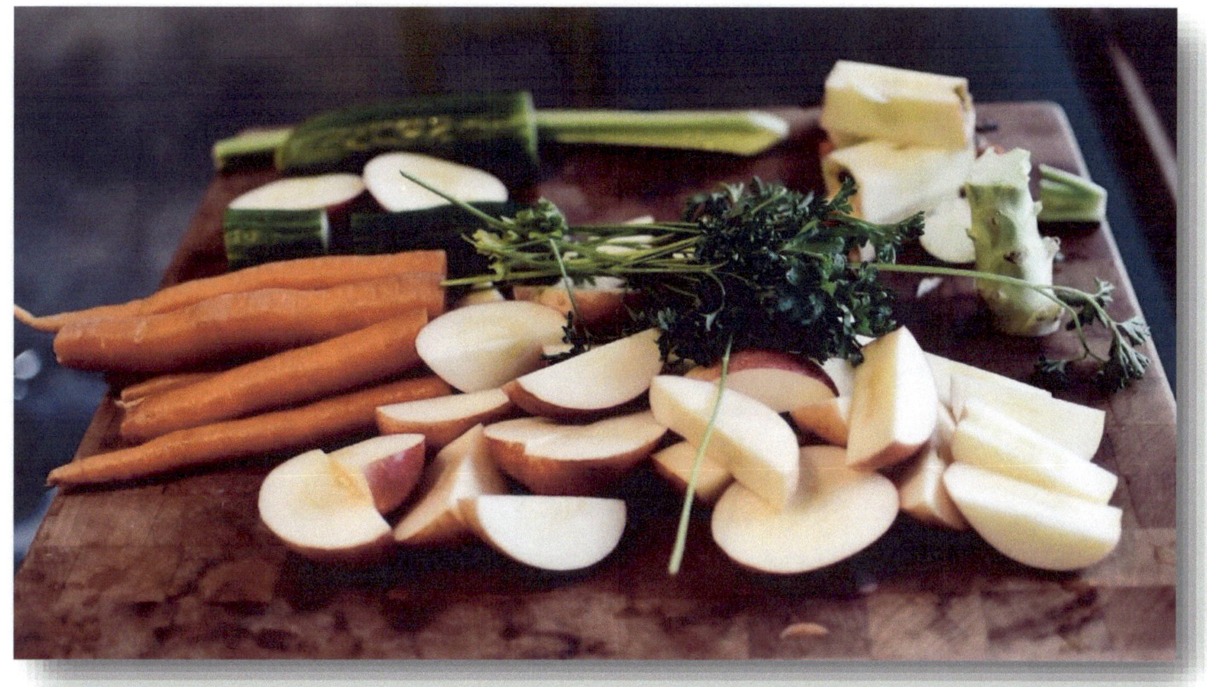

Published by:

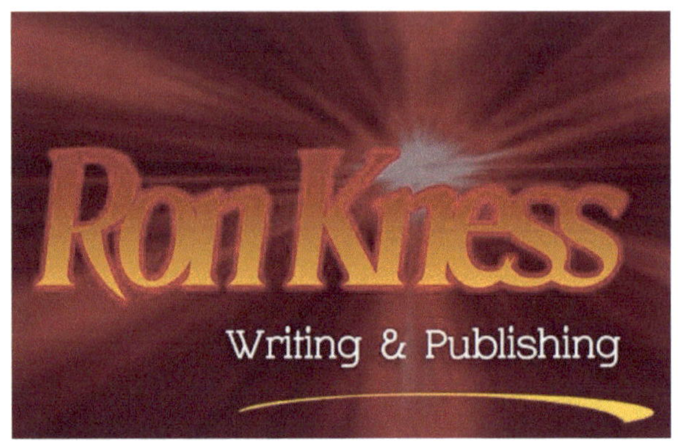

Ron Kness

San Tan Valley, AZ

United States of America

ISBN: 9781687230430

Disclaimer

We hope you enjoy reading this publication; however, we do suggest you read our disclaimer.

All the material written in this document is provided for informational purposes only and is general in nature.

Every person is a unique individual and what has worked for some or even many may not work for you. Any information perceived as advice must be considered in light of your own particular set of circumstances.

The author or person sharing this information does not assume any responsibility for the accuracy or outcome of your use of the content.

Every attempt has been made to provide well researched and up to date content at the time of writing. Now all the legalities have been taken care of, please enjoy the content.

Introduction

Due to the exponential increase in diagnosed cases of Type 2 diabetes, awareness of diabetes in a general sense has become widespread. In spite of this, there is no shortage of misinformation and misunderstanding about diabetes, including similarities and differences among the different types.

Depending on the type, diet can play a significant part in cause, prevention and especially management of the condition. A person suffering from diabetes, by necessity, must become more aware of the food they consume, especially food that spikes their blood sugar level.

Different diets and dietary protocols become much more than fleeting choices; for diabetics, they are truly lifestyle choices.

The ketogenic diet is one which has gained acceptance by many sufferers and medical practitioners. However, it is also a subject which has become a victim of misunderstanding.

This report explains what the ketogenic diet is and how it can be of help to many diabetics. It also has chapters on ketoacidosis, which will be very helpful in clearing up common misunderstandings between that dangerous condition and ketosis, which is a natural and mostly beneficial result of ketogenic dieting.

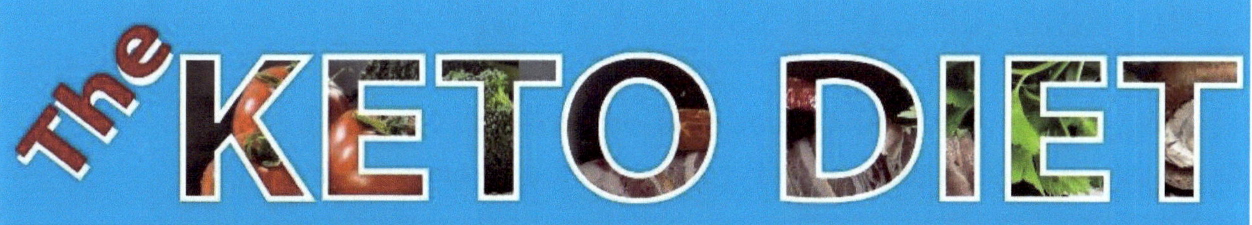

What is a Ketogenic Diet?

Sometimes referred to simply as "keto", this is a type of diet that involves the drastic reduction of carbohydrates and encourages increased intake of foods that are high in fat content.

This drastic reduction of carbohydrate intake puts the body into a state called "ketosis". This is when the body is forced to burn fat as a source of fuel, instead of glucose.

A very low-carb diet puts your body in a ketosis state. Fats will be turned into ketones inside the liver to supply the energy requirements of the brain and body.

The reduction in carb intake also provides lowered levels of blood sugar and subsequent need for insulin, which positively affects health in many areas.

Is the Ketogenic Diet Safe for Diabetics?

According to the American Diabetes Association, in 2015, over 30 million Americans had diabetes. This staggering number equates to about 9.4% of the population.

And even worse, diabetes was the 7th leading cause of death in the United States in 2015.

In recent years the ketogenic diet has received a lot of attention. Originally created to help combat epilepsy in pediatric patients, the ketogenic diet gained much more popularity as people noticed dramatic weight loss.

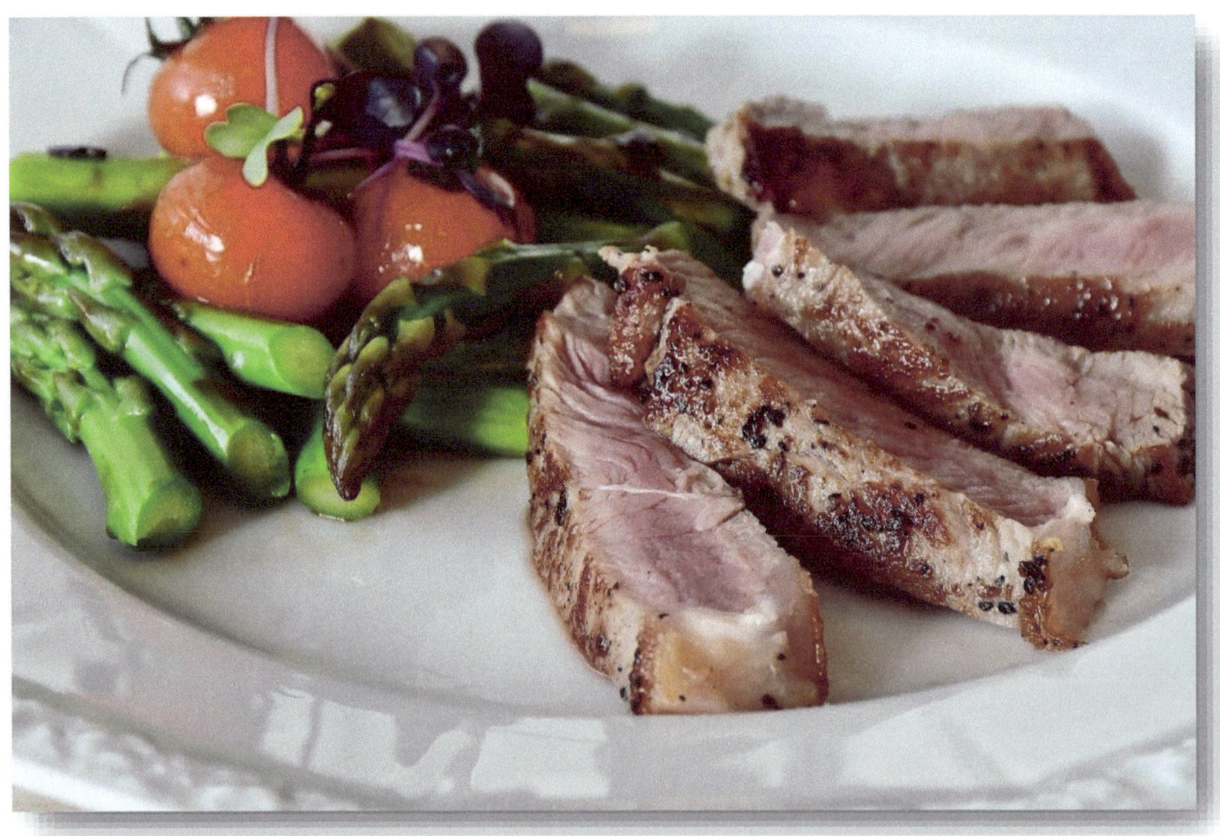

It has also been shown to help with chronic pain issues, fibromyalgia, arthritis, IBS, cholesterol, and blood pressure, to name a few. So, why wouldn't the ketogenic diet be beneficial for those people battling diabetes? Let's take a closer look.

What is Diabetes?

First, we need to cover some ground on diabetes in general. Glucose is the body's preferred source of fuel. When we eat, especially foods high in carbs and sugars, the body uses what it needs for fuel and stores the rest as fat.

The pancreas produces insulin to regulate glucose spikes in the bloodstream.

- Type 1 diabetes is diagnosed usually in adolescence or early adulthood and is characterized by insufficient insulin production which eventually turns into the inability to produce insulin at all.

  About 5% of all diabetics are Type 1 and it is known to be hereditary along with other factors still unexplained. Type 1 is usually treated with insulin injections.

- Type 2 diabetes can be diagnosed at any time and is characterized by insulin resistance. The body does not respond to insulin properly and eventually, slows the insulin production down. Most Type 2 diabetes is lifestyle-related.

  Obesity and inactivity have been linked to Type 2 diabetes. Diet, exercise, oral medication and injectable insulin are all ways to treat Type 2 diabetes with insulin injections being the last resort.

Can the Ketogenic Diet Help?

The short answer is *most probably, with some caveats*. Before attempting any dietary changes, it is imperative to consult ones' primary care provider and discuss options.

Dealing with diabetes is oftentimes tricky and depends a great deal on food choices. Without proper supervision, the results could be devastating.

Being in a state of nutritional ketosis should not be confused with diabetic ketoacidosis.

Nutritional ketosis is achieved when carbohydrates are restricted which causes the body to produce ketones from body fat to use as an alternate fuel. A healthy range of ketones is 0.1 mmol/liter to 1.5 mmol/liter.

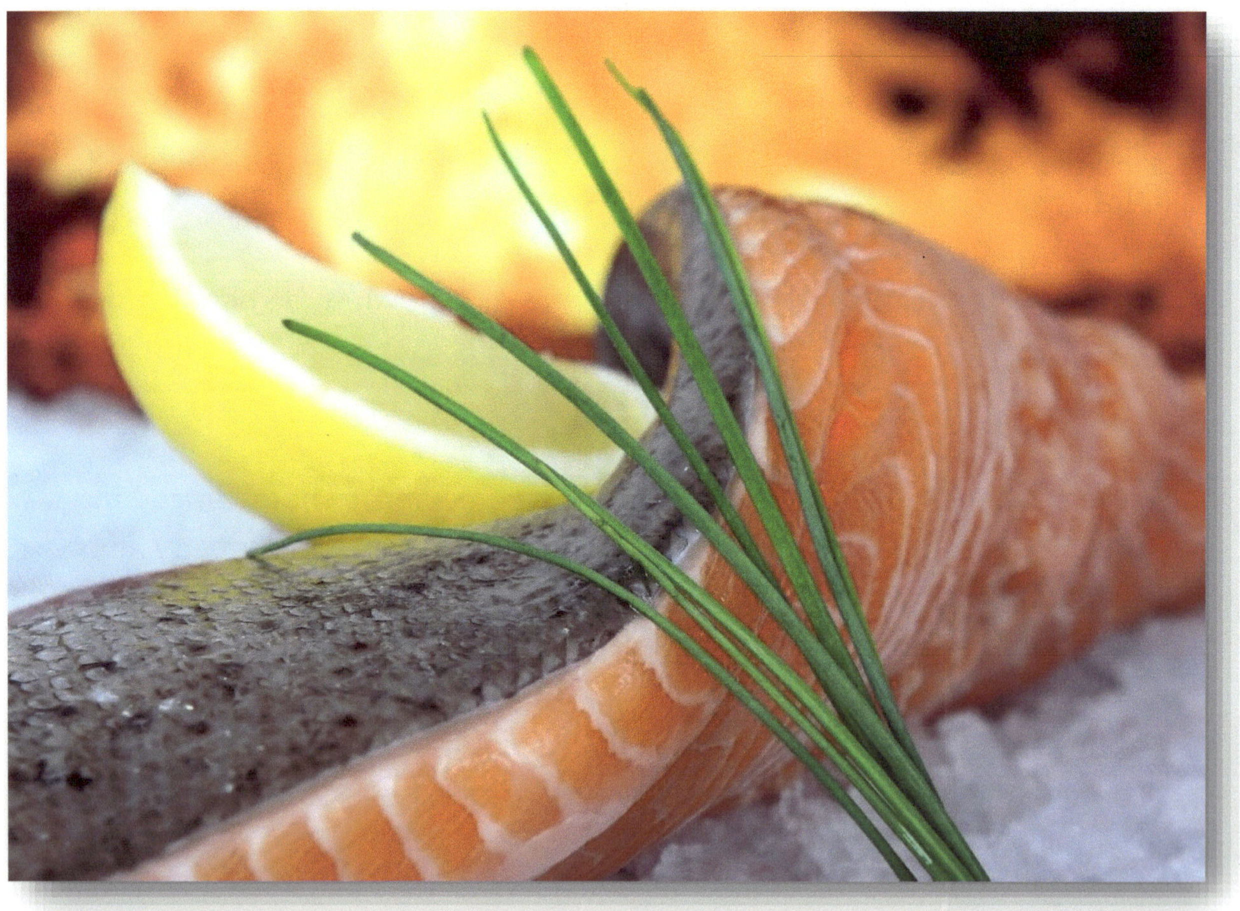

In diabetic ketoacidosis (DKA), the ketone range is 1.6 mmol/liter to more than 3.0 mmol/liter. DKA affects mostly type 1 diabetics when the lack of insulin production allows blood glucose to get extremely high.

Keto and Type 2 diabetes

In the most general terms, the ketogenic diet is safe for Type 2 diabetics. It's still good to check with one's primary physician prior to dietary changes since diabetes is so sensitive to foods containing sugar/carbs.

When in a state of nutritional ketosis, the body is using ketones for fuel, instead of sugar/glucose.

Therefore, blood sugar levels are naturally lower than eating a diet rich in carbohydrates. In turn, less insulin is required to regulate blood sugar levels. And in an insulin resistant body, this is good news.

With better controlled blood glucose levels and weight loss, diabetes becomes more manageable and could even go into remission.

The key though, is continuing this "diet" as a lifestyle and not a temporary fix.

Keto and Type 1 Diabetes

Because a Type 1 diabetic has the inability to produce insulin, the ketogenic diet needs constant and diligent monitoring. Glucose is basically trapped in the bloodstream and can't be deposited to the cells without medication.

And if carbohydrates are limited, there is less glucose produced, which means the potential for lower blood sugar levels and less spiking. Some might find it easier to have glucose tablets on hand for low blood sugar than relying on insulin injections for increased blood glucose levels.

There is no cure for diabetes, but it can be managed. With the ketogenic diet, the need for medication will likely rapidly decrease. There have been several studies done on the ketogenic diet in diabetes Type 2 proving its efficacy.

To date, the research on Type 1 is still very limited. As always, consult the doctor prior to altering diabetes treatment and dietary modifications.

Can the Ketogenic Diet Help Reverse Kidney Disease in Diabetics?

Little known fact: The ketogenic diet has been around for over 100 years. Originally developed for treating epilepsy in pediatric patients, in the 1970s the ketogenic way of eating took the diet world by storm because of its rapid weight loss properties.

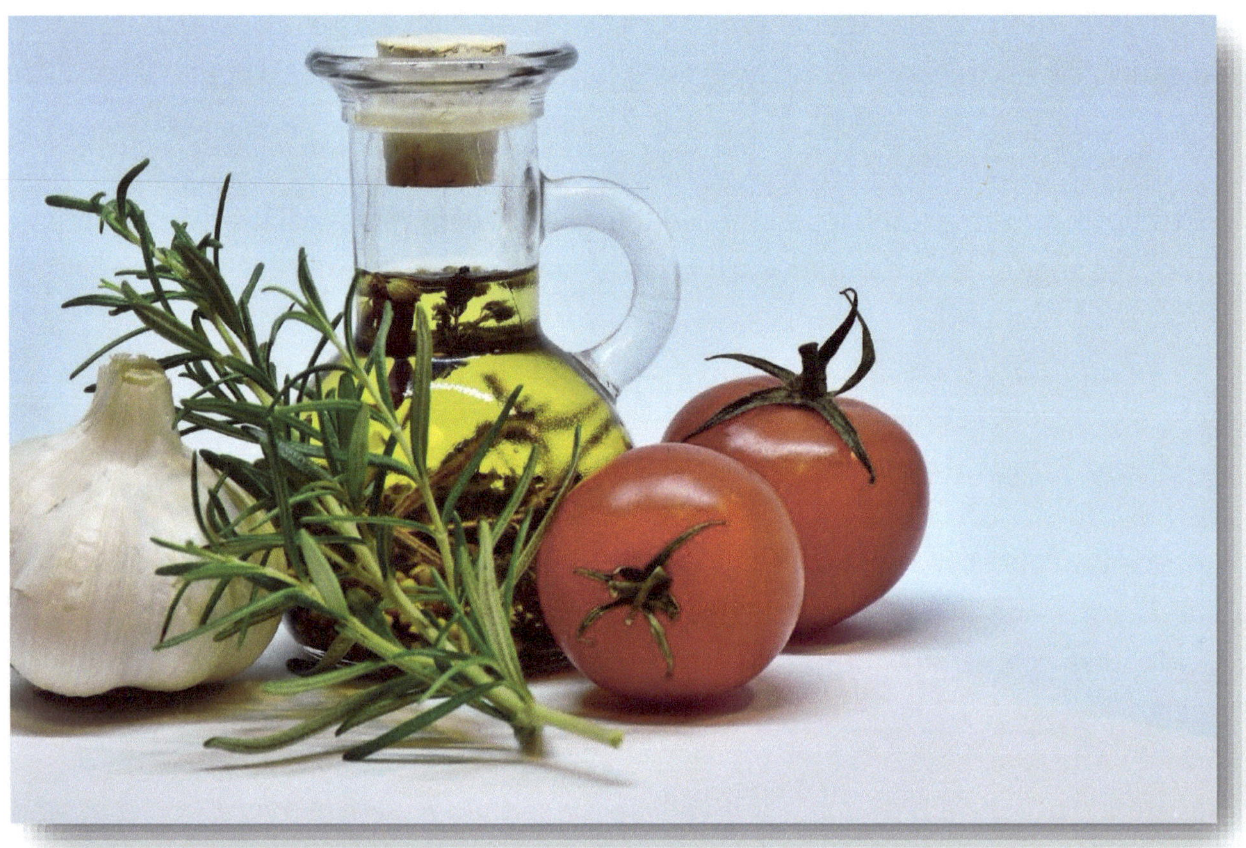

Since then, those enjoying keto-life have been under the microscope so to speak, as new developments in the ketogenic diet have come to light. For instance, when done properly, the ketogenic diet can help lessen chronic pain, lower blood pressure, lower bad cholesterol while bringing the good cholesterol up, and even help manage diabetes.

So, if diabetes control is on the list of advantages for following the ketogenic diet, does that also mean it's capable of reversing kidney disease caused by diabetes?

That would be exciting news for those with end-stage kidney disease facing dialysis, kidney transplant or even stem cell transplant for life-saving treatments.

The long and short of it is, animal research has indicated some promising developments and shocking results. As of yet, there is no official study on humans. However, if the hypotheses ring true, the future is looking much brighter for diabetics with kidney disease.

Ketogenic Fuel vs. Glucose Metabolism

In the ketogenic diet, ketones are produced because of the lack of carbohydrates. It's providing an alternate fuel source for itself to sustain organ function. Pretty ingenious.

The body naturally prefers carbohydrates for fuel, which is then converted into glucose. Using glucose for energy is called glucose metabolism.
In a diabetic, the obvious problem is how the body treats glucose spikes.

Insulin production problems (Type 1 diabetes) and insulin resistance once produced (Type 2 diabetes) leave glucose wandering around in the bloodstream wreaking havoc on the kidneys and other organs. One analogy is the glucose is like small glass shards that cut-up the inside of veins and arteries.

Could Ketogenic Fuel Be the Answer?

In the absence of glucose metabolism, one might assume the kidneys aren't being overworked and underpaid. The kidneys are responsible for filtering the bloodstream, which, in a diabetic, is infiltrated with unmetabolized glucose. Eventually, kidney cells can be damaged by so much stress.

With the ketogenic diet, glucose metabolism isn't even a notion. Ketones are used for energy, thus relieving the kidneys of undue stress and essentially allowing them to repair themselves.

Doctors and researchers are suggesting a month or two on the ketogenic diet is ample time for reversal of kidney disease in a diabetic.

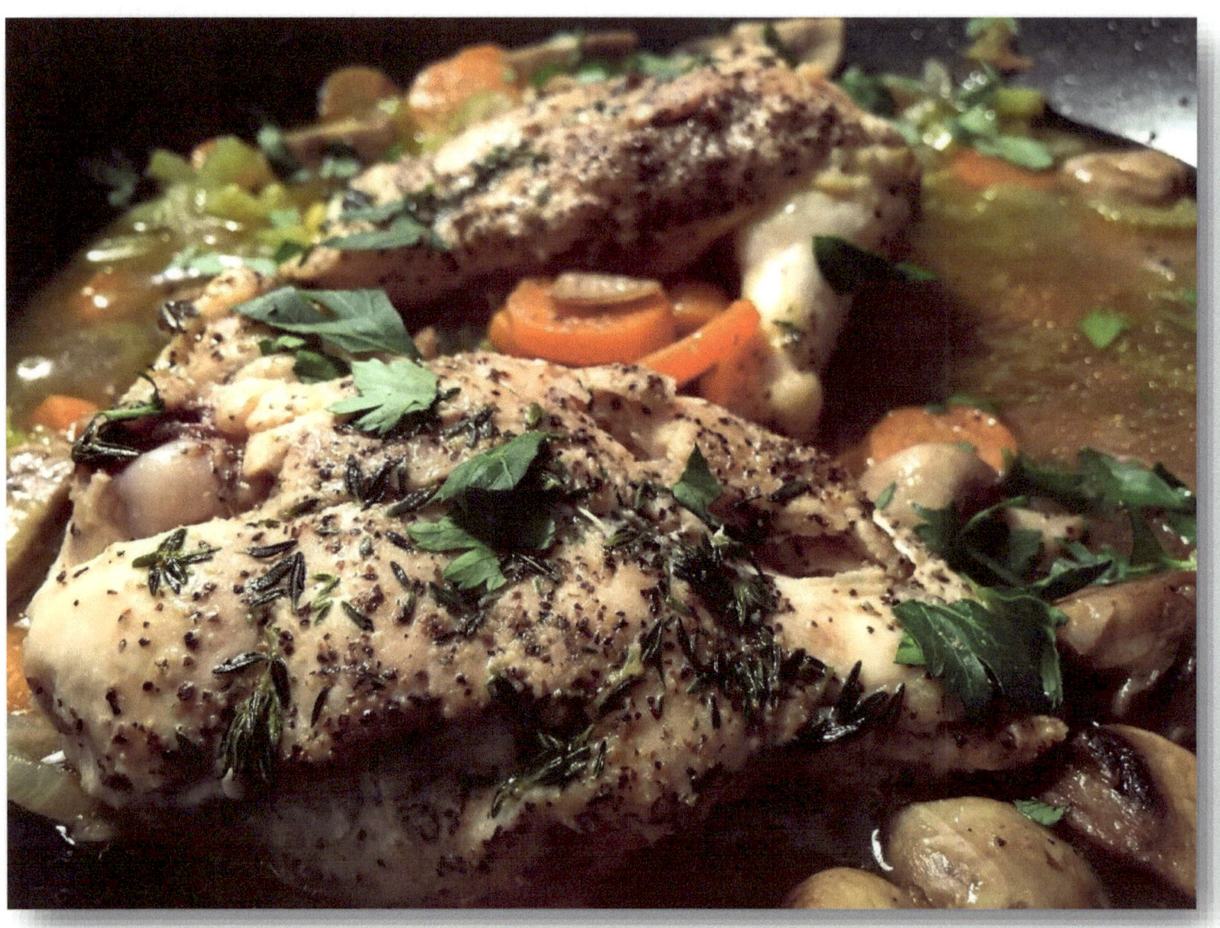

A Study on Mice

Researchers from Mount Sinai School of Medicine published a study, Reversal of Diabetic Nephropathy by a Ketogenic Diet, in the April 2011 issue of **PLoS ONE** claiming,
"… the ketogenic diet, a specialized high-fat, low-carbohydrate diet, may reverse impaired kidney function in people with Type 1 and Type 2 diabetes. "

If reading a scientific study filled with chemical equations and seemingly unpronounceable words doesn't sound like fun, take a look at the recap below:

The study was conducted on mice, all of which were genetically altered to develop Type 1 or Type 2 diabetes. The mice were then allowed to develop kidney failure, or diabetic nephropathy. The mice were split into two groups; the experiment and the control group.

The experiment group received the ketogenic diet while the control group received the standard high carbohydrate diet. After just eight weeks, mice given the ketogenic diet had reversed their kidney disease.

What Does This Mean for Humans

This is where things get hairy. There hasn't been any reported development on this theory in the last seven years, which only makes one wonder. Is there no funding for such an incredible, potentially life-saving therapy?

Or is "big pharma" conducting studies to create yet another money-making miracle pill? It's anyone's guess at this point.

The study proved the hypothesis that diet alone can reverse kidney disease in mice, however the question of how far advanced the disease can be and still see results from the ketogenic diet is still unanswered.

Some scientists believe advanced kidney disease and those already on dialysis are not going to see the same results. In looking at the big picture, this is astounding news for diabetics with kidney disease. Reversal of kidney disease by diet alone might even replace dialysis completely.

Which will undoubtedly bring on a plethora of questions for the ketogenic diet and its seemingly miraculous properties. Can it heal other neurological diseases? Retinopathy? Restless leg syndrome? Neuropathy? Time will only tell!

Long Term Effects of Following the Ketogenic Diet

The ketogenic diet is getting all sorts of attention as of late, there's no doubt about it. But is this just a fad diet or a long-term way of eating?

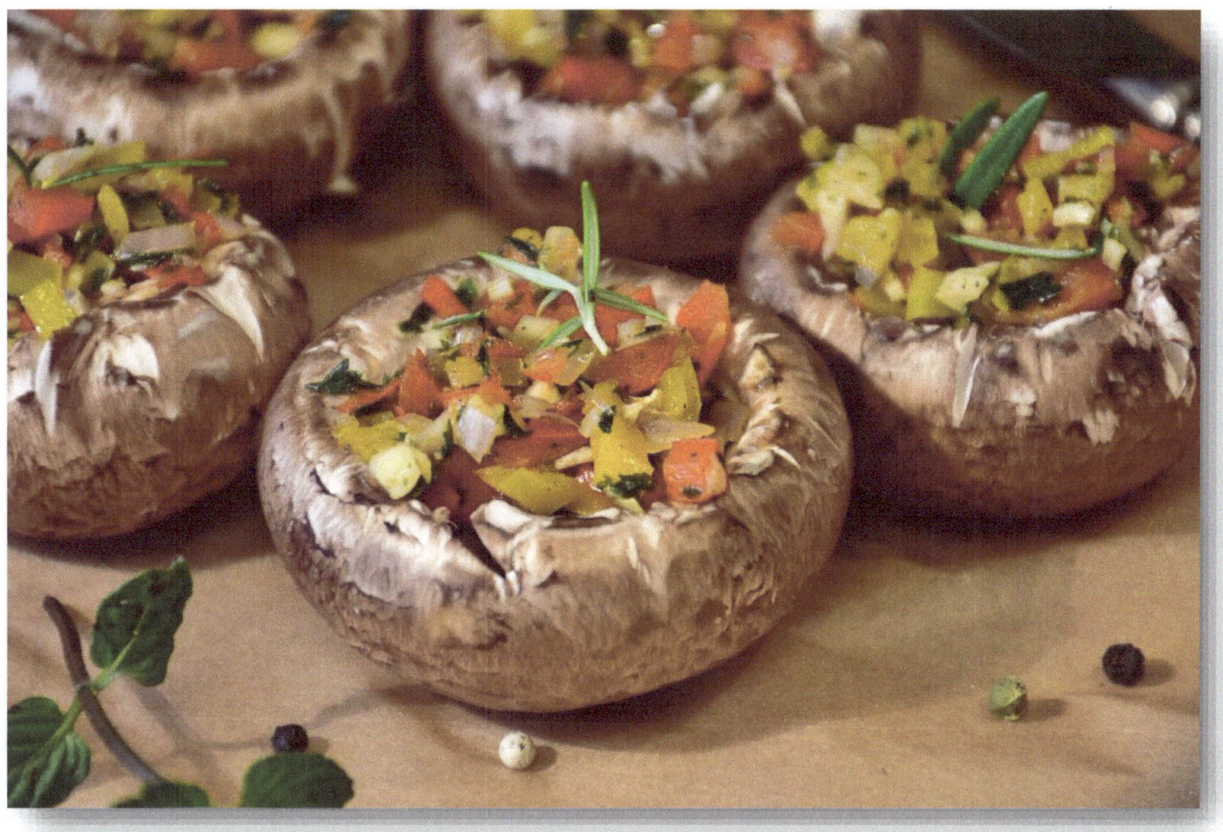

Most likely every human being concerned about their health has heard of the ketogenic diet and how incredibly fast weight melts away, but there are several other long-term effects, both benefits and risks, people should know before jumping in headfirst.

Unfortunately, the jury is still out on many long-term effects of the ketogenic diet due to a lack of clinical research.

The Good

Weight loss is probably the most popular reason people start a ketogenic diet. Dropping weight is very rapid for some and for others it may take a bit of time to achieve weight loss goals. Because of the decrease in weight, many people see improved cardiovascular health, less difficulty with chronic pain and fibromyalgia, as well as decreased symptoms of polycystic ovarian syndrome (PCOS).

In addition, once keto-adapted, the body is effectively using fat for energy instead of glucose-based fuel thus blood glucose levels are generally better controlled. This is especially advantageous for those battling with diabetes or hypoglycemia.

And, because better sources of food are on the menu, cholesterol levels generally improve. Along with mental alertness and cognitive performance. Speaking of food sources, another benefit of the ketogenic diet is the lack of cravings.

Sugar products seem to taste much sweeter than before and less desirable. Carb cravings aren't usually a problem after a while either.

The Bad

Of course, it isn't all sunshine and roses. Many people report having bad breath, foul-smelling urine and even a different perspiration odor. This is caused from the acid byproduct of ketones being excreted and typically goes away after complete adaptation to the ketogenic diet.

Dehydration is a worry for some as well. Drinking a prescribed amount of water daily isn't really necessary with the ketogenic diet like it is with other diet plans. The body simply doesn't retain as much water. Drink to thirst. That's the ticket.

Headaches, lethargy and the dreaded keto-flu are other "bad" effects and will undoubtedly continue long-term if not properly addressed. The long and short of it is an electrolyte imbalance.

Sodium, magnesium and potassium should be tracked to make sure daily allowances are achieved and supplemented when necessary.

Let's talk poop. Another long-term effect for some is constipation. There is a difference though, in not pooping and constipation. With the ketogenic diet, much of the food eaten is being used by the body, thus less excrement is normal. Constipation, on the other hand, is painful and avoidable in most cases by increasing fiber.

The Ugly

There's not much to report on by reliable sources regarding ugly long-term effects of the ketogenic diet. Naysayers and nonbelievers spout out the potential for kidney damage and kidney stones, but the truth is this is more than likely a problem for those with a pre-existing kidney disorder or predisposition for kidney stones.

Gallstones is another one some have claimed. From a medical perspective, gallstones are a result of an inactive gallbladder. The gallbladder's main job is the flush fat, so by feeding it fat (good fat, not bad fat) it revs the motor and starts working.

Now, if someone has enjoyed a low-fat diet for a good while and then jumps into keto where fat is abundant, the gallbladder gets going and tries to flush out the sludge it's been holding while just sitting there doing nothing.

In cases like this, yes, gallstones might be an issue... but this isn't really a long-term term thing as long as the gallbladder stays awake and on the job.

The worst characteristic one can really say about the ketogenic diet long-term is the ability to sustain such a restrictive way of eating. There are times and circumstances when eating keto-friendly isn't an option.

Those who travel a lot for work or even going to a friend's cookout might find the ketogenic diet a bit cumbersome. That's where preparedness comes into play.

Think outside the box. Bring a keto-friendly dish to the cookout and make sure there is food on hand that doesn't require refrigeration while traveling; like flavored tuna packets, avocados, jerky, nuts, etc.

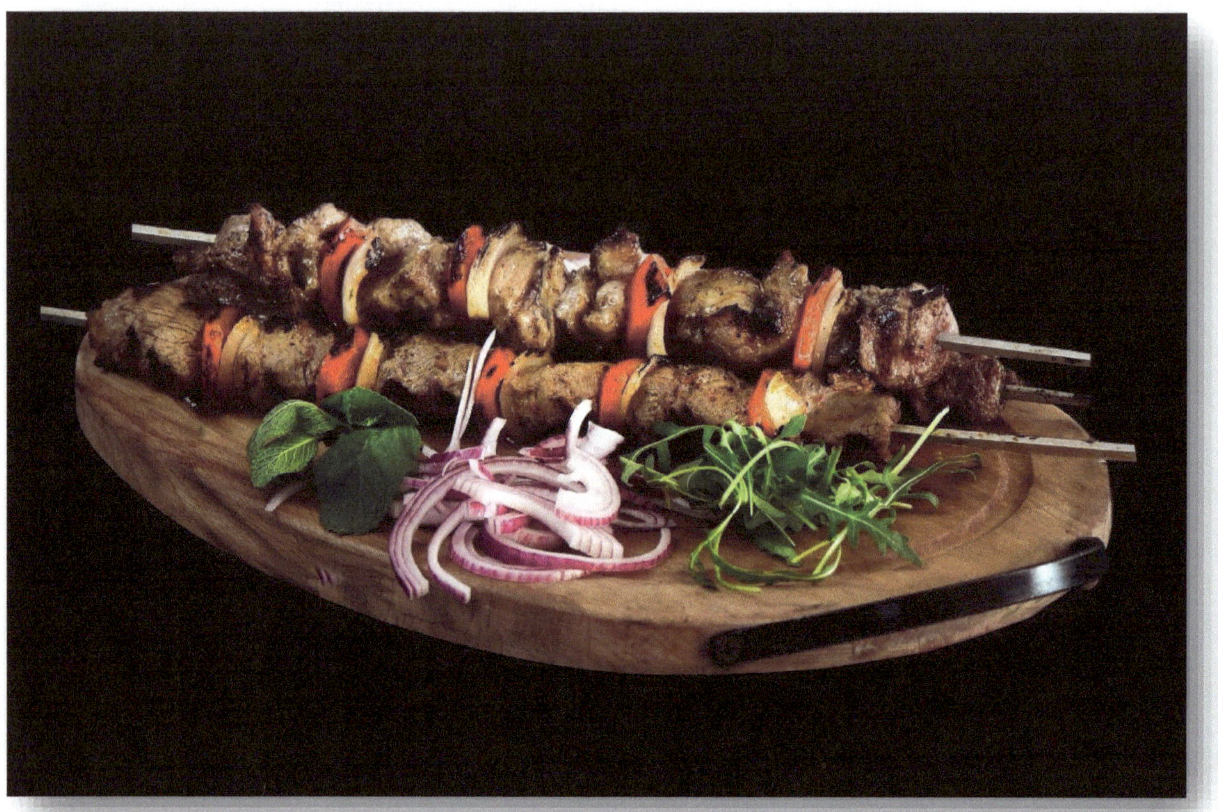

The Future

The ketogenic diet isn't just for weight loss and secondary benefits therein. There is research being conducted now on treatment for different types of cancers. It is believed certain cancers feed on glucose. The concept is by eliminating glucose, cancer cells starve to death.

Researchers are also hard at work with benefits of the ketogenic diet in those with Alzheimer's Disease and even Autism Disorder. If it is effective in reducing seizures by 50% of epilepsy patients who have given it a whirl, wouldn't it be likely other neurologic disorders could also benefit from this way of eating? The sky is the limit.

The ketogenic diet is very simple. Literally. Get rid of the toxins and chemicals and keep things as natural as possible. It tastes better and it's better for the body. Long ago, people survived off the land and didn't have boxed meals or processed foods.

Guess what else they didn't have… Diabetes, hypertension, high cholesterol, morbid obesity… The ketogenic diet is all about getting back to the basics. Getting back to what works. And it does work!

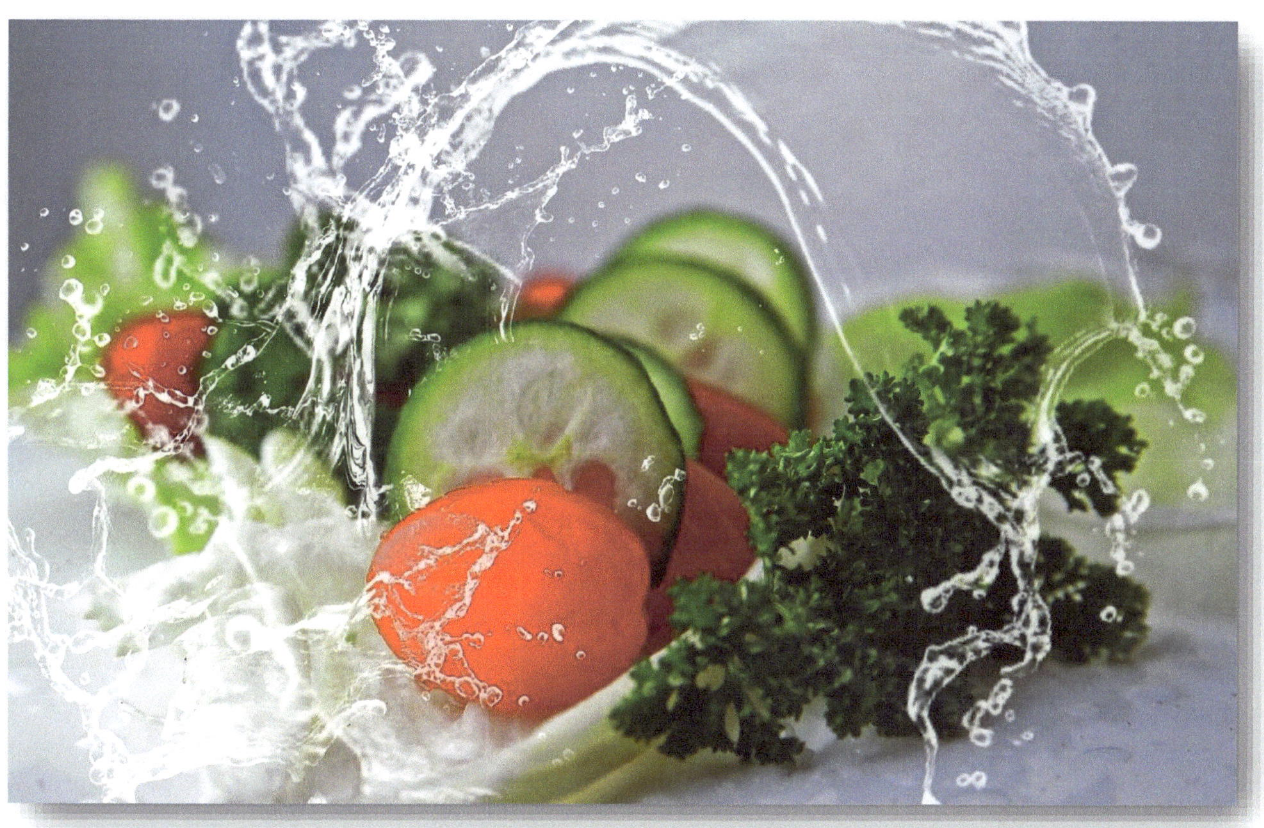

What Happens When You Have Diabetic Ketoacidosis?

Diabetic ketoacidosis (DKA) is a condition affecting those with diabetes mellitus when the blood becomes too acidic. It primarily strikes those with Type 1 and occurs much less often in those with Type 2 diabetes.

One should seek immediate medical attention if the signs and symptoms of DKA are present and not attempt to treat this at home. This condition can be life-threatening.

Keto + Acid + Osis

In examining the word "ketoacidosis" one would not assume insulin is the main culprit, however a lack of insulin in the bloodstream is, without a doubt, the primary cause. DKA would not be such a devastating and terrifying event if insulin was properly produced and/or absorbed into the cells.

Keto – When there is an inadequate supply of glucose (sugars/carbohydrates) to use for fuel, the liver responds by producing *ketones* as an alternate fuel source.

Acid – Ketones are broken down for energy and *acid* is the byproduct.

Osis – Medical term for a "condition" or "process".

The Perfect Storm

Diabetics commonly refer to diabetic ketoacidosis as the perfect storm. It can come on fast and furious, without much warning, and even happen to the most careful diabetics religiously monitoring blood glucose levels.

Part 1: Lack of insulin causes which causes elevated glucose levels.

As mentioned above, insulin (the lack of) is the real villain in this saga. And lack of insulin in the body could happen for any number of reasons:

- Illness, infection and personal stressors. During times of great stress on the body, stress hormones are produced. Even if there is enough insulin, the stress hormones block insulin from doing its job.

- Missed/Skipped injections. Occasionally, missing a dose of insulin isn't going to create a state of diabetic ketoacidosis. However, missed long-acting insulin doses or repeated skipped doses of regular insulin could turn the tables.

- Ketones could be produced by intentional lack of carbohydrates, such as with the ketogenic diet. If the body is producing ketones at a rate which exceeds the body's capability to use and excrete what's not used, DKA might be right around the corner.

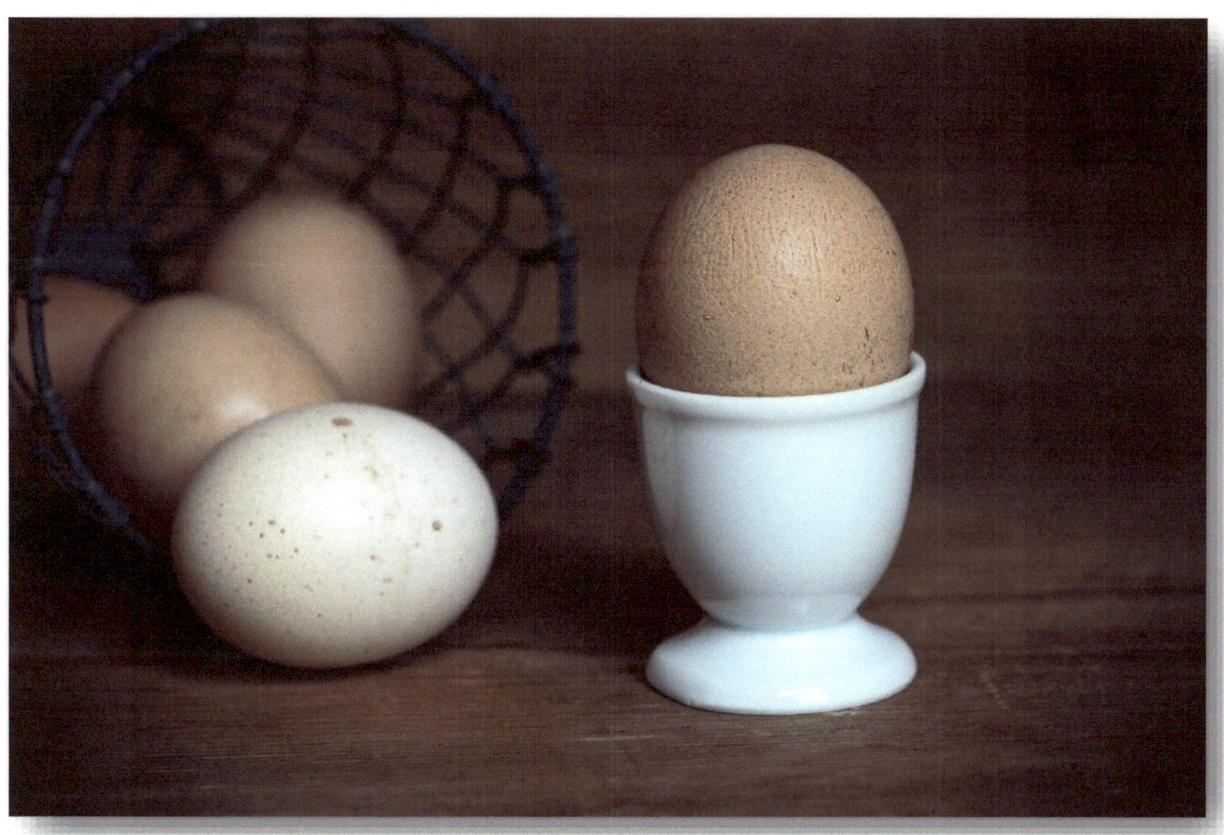

- Poor absorption. Diabetics may need to switch injection sites.

- Spoiled insulin. Obviously, expired insulin shouldn't be used, but proper storage and avoiding extreme temperatures needs to be avoided as well.

- Insulin pump malfunction. Any interruption in delivery or absorption could lead to DKA.

Part 2: Elevated ketone levels.

Ketone production, whether intentional or not, can lead to higher levels of acid in the blood. An unbalanced pH level can be toxic. Monitoring ketones in a diabetic is essential, especially when a factor in part 1 of the perfect storm is in play. Ketones can be tested by urine, blood and even breath.

Part 3: The symptoms.

The symptoms of diabetic ketoacidosis are much like that of the flu or food poisoning. In fact, they are so similar, diabetics oftentimes will try to self-medicate with insulin and fluids and unnecessarily put themselves at risk for kidney failure, heart attack, coma and death.

Among the most common symptoms are:

- Dehydration
- Intense thirst
- Dry mouth
- Fruity-smelling breath, but in a bad way
- Headache
- Muscle aches
- Nausea and vomiting
- Upset stomach or stomach pain
- Flushed skin
- Dry skin

More extreme symptoms are:

- Vomiting more than twice in a two-hour period
- Confusion
- Word-finding difficulty
- Heart palpitations
- Shortness of breath
- Extreme lethargy

To recap, the perfect storm is an event disrupting insulin production and/or absorption, elevated glucose levels, elevated ketone levels and any number of flu-like symptoms.

Treatment for DKA

The preferred treatment is fluids, electrolyte replacement and insulin. Like any other hospital stay there should be a team of medical professionals overseeing one's care, performing exams and tests, ordering the appropriate regimen for the circumstances and education to prevent further episodes.

Diabetic ketoacidosis can happen to any diabetic, even the veterans. In fact, many go to the emergency room and DKA uncovers a diagnosis of diabetes. The best defense is education for the diabetic *and* those close to them. Sometimes people feel a trip to emergency services is unwarranted and need to be urged to seek help.

It can't be stressed enough: DKA requires professional medical help and when left untreated can lead to kidney damage, heart attack, coma and death. The quicker medical attention is sought, the better the chances of a quick recovery.

Difference Between Ketosis and Diabetic Ketoacidosis

There's no denying the similarities in the words, ketosis and ketoacidosis, but their definitions aren't nearly the same. The main concept behind the ketogenic diet is achieving and maintaining a state of nutritional ketosis.

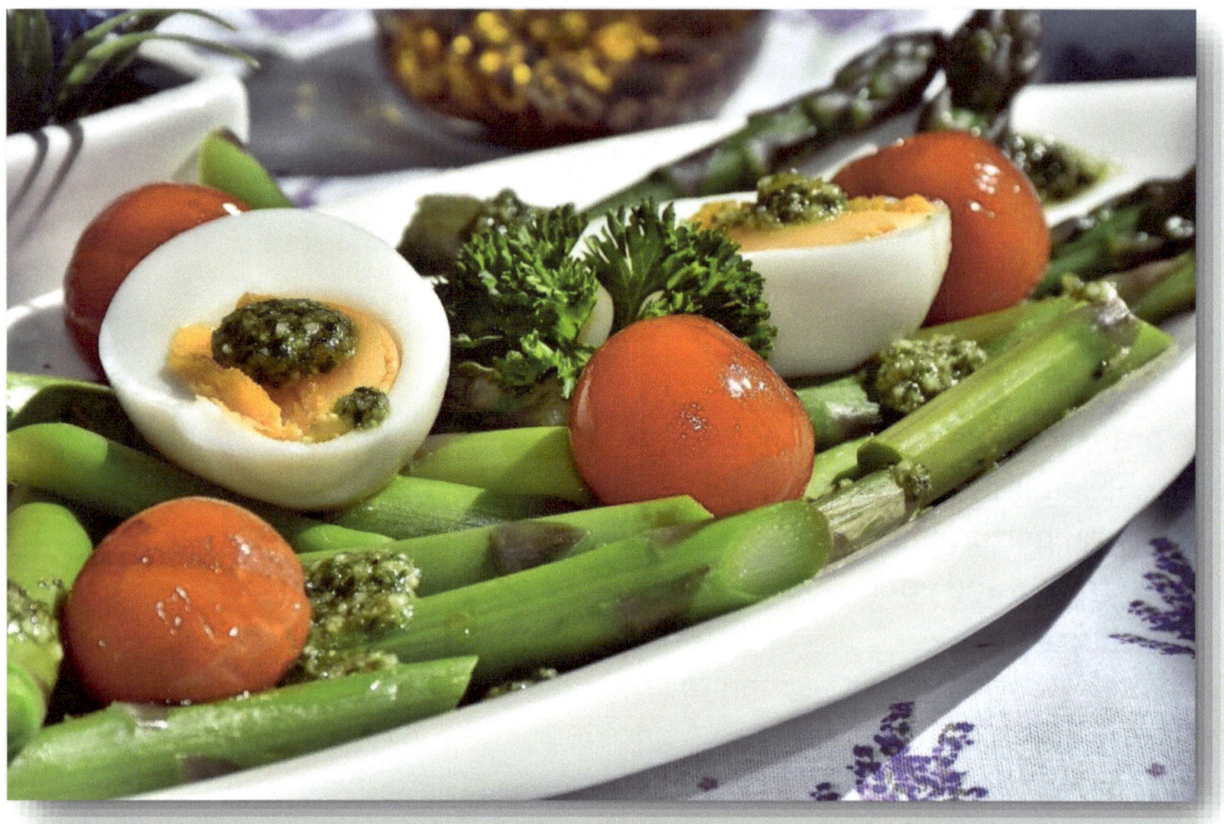

Ketoacidosis is a dangerous and life-threatening condition typically in diabetics with uncontrolled insulin and an extremely elevated blood ketone level.

Many people shy away from the ketogenic diet due to a lack of understanding of these two words. Admittedly, they are easily confused. Even health care professionals sometimes assume a patient is referring to diabetic ketoacidosis (DKA) just at the mention of ketosis.

Don't get offended or think the doctor flunked medical school. They are trained to try and make sense of patients who may not be very knowledgeable when it comes to medical terminology.

Ketosis Defined

Nutritional ketosis, as stated above, is the first goal of the ketogenic diet. The human body uses glucose, which is provided by sugars/carbohydrates, as its first choice for energy generation.

When carbohydrates are limited, as in the ketogenic diet, the body adapts and begins to use stored fats (fatty acids released from the cells and converted to ketones in the liver).

Generally, it takes up to 48 hours to achieve a state of nutritional ketosis and could take several weeks for the body to fully adapt. It should be noted though, as soon as glucose is available, it will immediately revert to that energy.

Ketoacidosis Defined

This unstable metabolic state is a complication of diabetes mellitus, predominantly type 1 and much less common in type 2, where the ketone level has gone way above and beyond the normal, healthy levels like in nutritional ketosis, *combined* with an elevated blood glucose level. The culprit for ketoacidosis is usually mismanagement of insulin therapy along with a poor diet.

Signs and Symptoms

Bad breath, somewhat like fermented fruit, is a good indication the body has achieved nutritional ketosis. The body breaks down ketones for fuel and a byproduct is acetone. The acetone is released via urine and funky breath.

Other signs could be lethargy and a flu-like stage, commonly called "keto-flu", which goes away with adaptation of the new energy source.

Ketoacidosis has a very different presentation:

- Frequent urination
- Extreme thirst, dry mouth
- Dehydration
- Nausea and/or vomiting
- Stomach pain
- Confusion
- Feeling short of breath

While ketoacidosis may also present with fermented fruit breath and feeling overly tired, the symptoms above are much more severe and require immediate medical attention.

Risk Factors

Nutritional ketosis is usually self-induced and done with purpose, for instance weight loss or for other medical reasons. It is a completely normal metabolic state and safe for most people.

The biggest risk factor for diabetic ketoacidosis is having diabetes Type 1. In fact, during the initial diagnosis of diabetes many patients are already in a state of DKA which is what led them to the doctor in the first place.

Other risk factors include alcoholism, drug abuse, missing one or more doses of insulin and improper diet. Also, some over-the-counter, prescription and illicit drugs may lessen the efficacy of normal insulin doses.

How Are the Two Diagnosed and Treated?

Blood Ketones: Normal to Moderate range is 0.6 to 1.5 mmol/L. High is 1.5 to 3.0 mmol/L. Anything over 3 mmol/L is considered dangerous.
Urine Ketones: 0.6 to 3.0 mmol/L is nutritional ketosis and 3 to 5 mmol/L is starvation ketosis.

Anything over 5 mmol/L is concerning for DKA if blood sugar is also elevated to greater than 250 mg/dL and one should seek medical attention immediately!

> *Over-the-counter blood ketone monitors can be purchased and is the most reliable detection method. Also available are urine strips and even breath monitors, however their results may not be as accurate.*

Diabetics usually remain in the low to moderate range for blood ketones on the ketogenic diet, safely and without much risk for ketoacidosis, as long as blood sugars are managed properly. Remember, both elevated ketones *and* elevated blood glucose levels indicate higher risk for DKA.

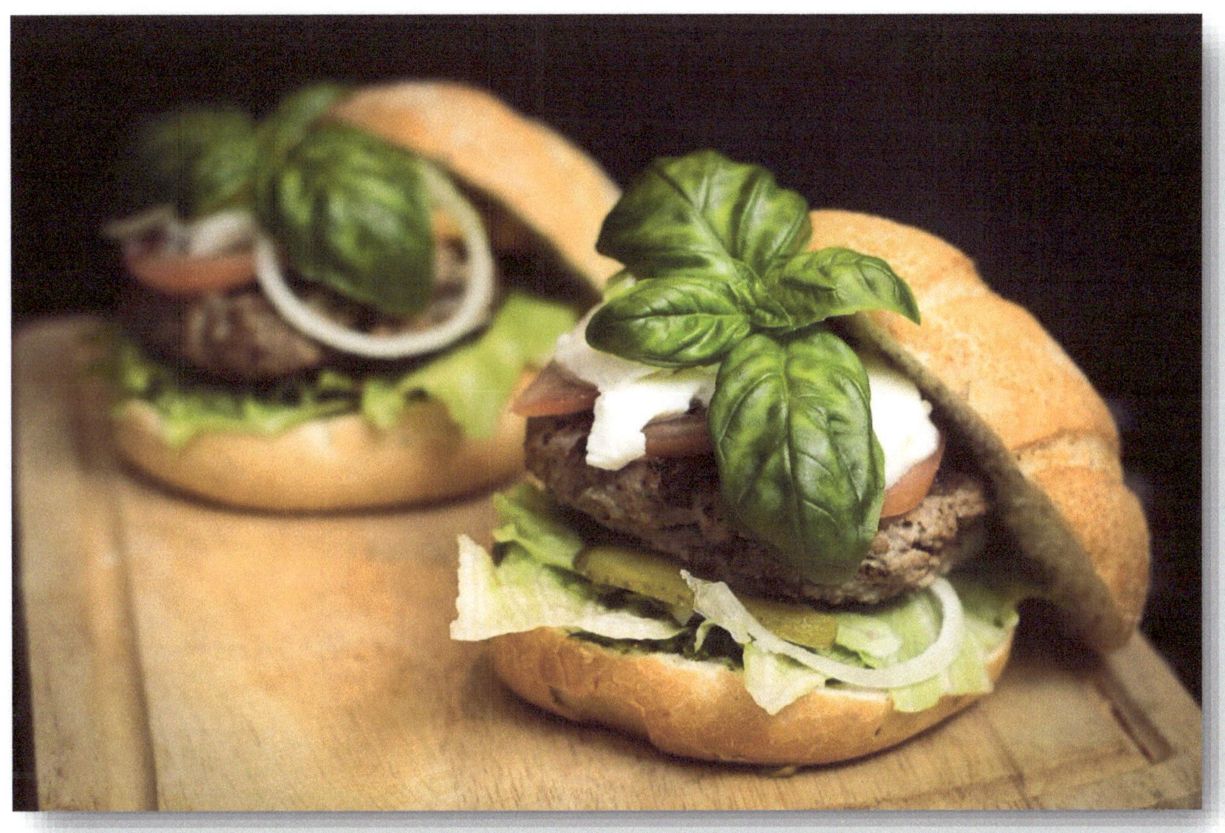

Doctors perform a physical exam, check ketone and blood sugar levels and ask a series of questions pertaining to symptom duration and severity, diabetes management or lack thereof, co-occurring illnesses or infections, increased stress, and if drugs or alcohol are on board.

Fluid and electrolyte replacement by mouth or intravenously along with subcutaneous or intravenous insulin are the modes of treatment for diabetic ketoacidosis.

Nutritional ketosis requires no treatment. If and when one no longer desires to be in a state of nutritional ketosis, reintroduction of carbohydrates is all it takes. The body automatically switches back to using glucose for fuel.

In summary, ketosis is a natural metabolic state where the body purposefully uses fats for fuel, enhances weight loss and has a number of other benefits for health and wellness.

Diabetic ketoacidosis is a potentially life-threatening unstable metabolic state usually caused by dysregulation of diabetes along with elevated ketone levels and requires immediate attention.

As always, diabetics should always consult with a primary care provider or diabetes management team prior to dietary changes. While the ketogenic diet is safe for most people, there are some circumstances where closer monitoring may be necessary.

Conclusion

Hopefully, this publication has cleared up much of the misunderstanding regarding the ketogenic diet, particularly as it relates to diabetics.

Correctly undertaken, the ketogenic diet will be of benefit to many diabetics, especially Type 2 sufferers.

Those with Type 1 diabetes can also employ the ketogenic diet, but must monitor the effects more closely. Of course, their condition demands they need to be constantly aware of their food consumption and its effects always.

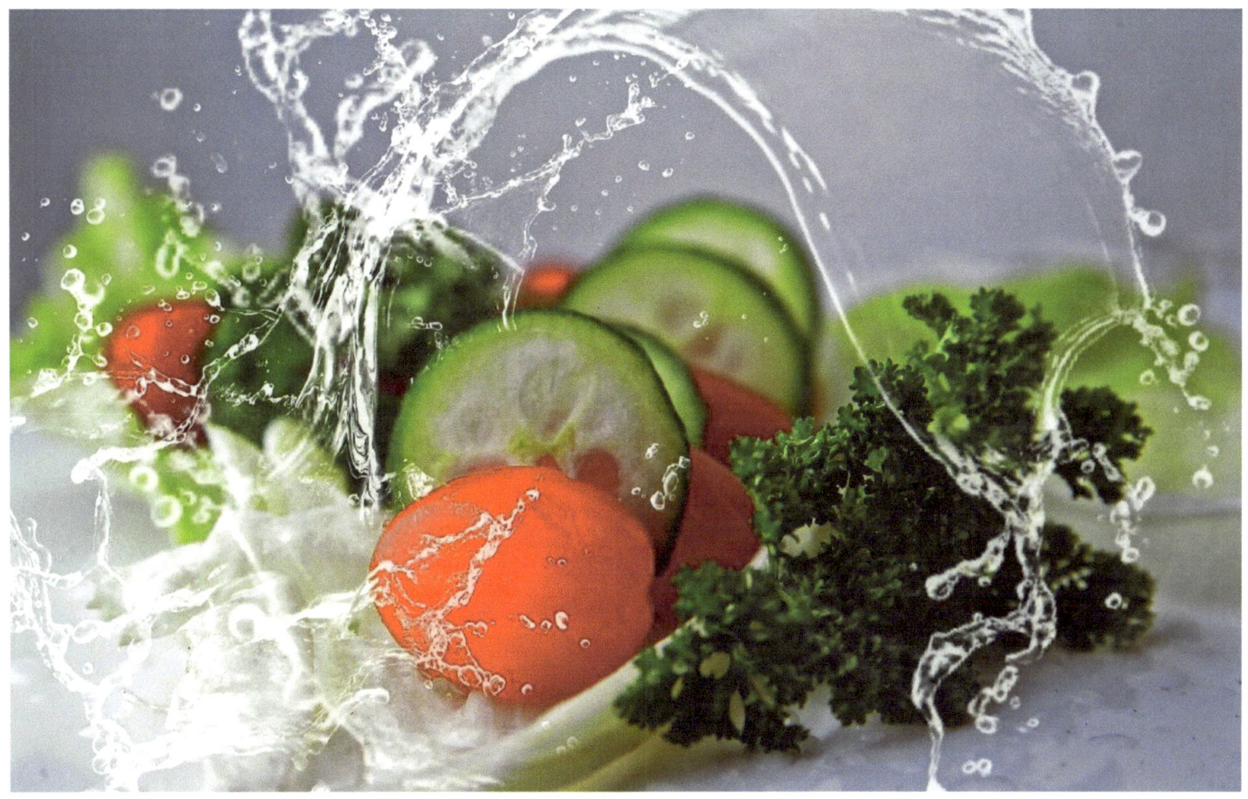

When dealing with the symptoms of diabetes, there is no one silver bullet, but the ketogenic diet, for most diabetics, is a good and healthy platform to start from.

About the Author

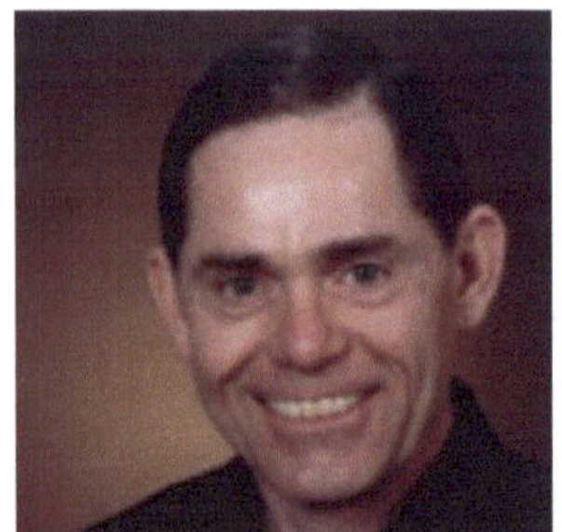 I have published numerous books on Amazon for Kindle and other publishing platforms. Both in electronic and POD formats.

While most of my books are on health and fitness in general, my topics of interest of late are leaning more toward aging baby boomers and the older population.

Besides my own writing, I also ghostwrite ebooks, books, reports, articles, blogs, email series for autoresponders and do Kindle conversions for clients on a variety of topics. Go to my website at http://ronknesswriting.com for more information or to submit a quote.

For a complete list of my published books, go to https://www.amazon.com/Ron-Kness/e/B0072M6PYO.

Today my wife and I are retired from our careers and live in San Tan Valley, AZ. I now write as a retirement business where you'll find me happily sitting in my office typing away on my laptop as I work on my next book or ghostwriting project . . . that is if we are not traveling on a cruise ship - our new-found mode of travel.